ORGANIC LIP BALMS

REJUVENATE, NOURISH AND PROTECT YOUR LIPS NATURALLY

Disclaimer and Terms of Use:

Effort has been made to ensure that the information in this book is accurate and complete, however, the author and the publisher do not warrant the accuracy of the information, text and graphics contained within the book due to the rapidly changing nature of science, research, known and unknown facts and internet. The Author and the publisher do not hold any responsibility for errors, omissions or contrary interpretation of the subject matter herein. This book is presented solely for motivational and informational purposes only.

Contents

Introduction

Whenever the cool and dry months come around, both men and women usually experience dry, chapped lips. The skin on the lips begins to peel, crack and hurt. So much so, that it feels like sandpaper. Nobody wants chapped lips, but the lack of moisture around your lips during these months makes this a common problem. However, there is an effective remedy to this problem: *Lip balms.*

Lip balms have been developed to help people keep their lips moisturized and prevent chapped lips. Some use it occasionally, while others on a daily basis, keeping the thinnest, driest, and most transparent tissue of your body, the lips, healthy. Although there are several kinds of lip balms available on the market today, it's important that you know not all of them are effective. Some are proven not to work at all, while there are others that contain ingredients that are harmful and addictive for your lips' sensitive skin.

That's why more people are moving to healthier and more natural alternative, which are organic lip balms!

Now, what you might be wondering is what's the difference? Well, the main difference between regular and organic lip balms is the way they are produced. Organic lip balms are completely free of pesticides, chemicals, and several other types of additives commonly found in regular lip balms, making them healthier and beneficial alternative. And that's exactly what this eBook is all about!

Not only will we provide you in-depth information regarding organic lip balms, you will also find some really useful organic lip balm recipes, which you can start applying straight away. So, do you want to rejuvenate, nourish and protect your lips as naturally as possible? Go through this eBook and get ready to bid farewell to your chapped lips once and for all!

Difference between Lip Balm & Lip Gloss

Lip balms and lip-gloss are two distinct lip care products, yet several people confuse one with the other. This is why it is imperative that we start the eBook by explaining the actual difference between the two products.

A lip balm (also called lip salve) is a wax-like substance that is applied to the lips topically in order to relieve and moisturize dry or chapped lips. Some medicated varieties are also used for the treatment of numerous lip conditions, such as Angular cheilitis, stomatitis, and cold sores.

The main purpose of lip balms is to provide the surface of your lip with an occlusive layer so that it can be protected from external exposure. Lip balms come in small cylinders or round jars and are usually applied using the fingers.

On the other hand, lip-gloss is a product that provides the lips a glossy luster, and sometimes a subtle color (depending on the type of lip-gloss you use). They are available in a soft solid or liquid form and should not be confused with lip balms, which generally have soothing or medicinal purposes. Lip-gloss comes in small cylindrical bottles with a doe foot applicator, or built-in lip brush.

While there is a huge difference between the two lip-care products, both have one common concern: *sharing them can lead to the transfer of some medical conditions or diseases.* Yes, unless you want to catch a nasty infection (which is unlikely), it is extremely important that you do not share your lip balm or lip-gloss with anybody.

Many people, particularly women, have the bad habit of sharing beauty products and though the gesture may be a good one, the result could be a contagious and painful infection.

So, now that we are on the same page about lip balms, let us move on to the next chapter where we will discuss the numerous benefits organic lip balms bring to the table.

The Benefits of Organic Lip Balms

Having chapped lips is undoubtedly an unpleasant experience, it hurts and burns, and it also looks unpleasant. Therefore, whether you are providing daily care to avoid them, or going through misery to remedy them, you will need to provide your lips with moisturizing nutrients. This is exactly when organic lip balms come in and provide your lips with the ingredients they require.

Organic lip balms have a lot to offer and to give you a better idea of that, in the following paragraphs; we have discussed the benefits of organic lip balms:

True Protection & Nutrition

Since organic lip balms are completely free from any chemical compounds, which are commonly found in synthetic lip balms, they will provide you 100% benefits without any detracting aspects. The most common natural ingredients used in organic lip balms are aloe Vera, beeswax, Shea butter, cocoa butter, olive oil, and jojoba essential oil.

Cocoa butter provides fragrant notes and moisturizing effects, while olive oil is loaded with antioxidants in the form of Vitamin C and Vitamin E. Aloe Vera in particular, is an essential ingredient in lip balms, as it provides a range of therapeutic benefits. It improves hydration by penetrating the skin of your lips and helps with the speedy recovery of chapped lips. It also believed that aloe vera stimulates the skin and assists cell growth.

This means that unlike regular and synthetic lip balms, organic lip balms will provide you true protection and nutrition, that too without the involvement of any side effects or detracting aspects whatsoever!

Protection against the Sun

You already might be hearing a lot about the dangers of excess sun exposure, but the statistics can still shock you. According to a study, around 90% of the 600,000 new skin cancer cases reported every year are caused by exposure to sunlight sun. Those are quite staggering figures!

Keeping this in mind, let's bring one important fact about your lips into attention: *they are one of the most vulnerable parts of the human body.*

Yes, since they are on our face, they are exposed to the sun almost every time you step outside, so much so, that even commonly used accessories such as hats, scarves and sunglasses, usually do not shade the lips. This is why it is extremely important that you are careful about sun exposure.

However, luckily there are lip balms available that provide sun protection as well. An ingredient, zinc oxide, is typically used in organic lip balms for this purpose, which provides your lips with full protection from harmful UVB and UVA rays. Therefore, whether you are on the slopes, at the beach or anywhere you need protection from the sun, you can rest assured organic lip balms will keep your lips healthy and happy.

Free From Chemicals & Additives

One of the biggest benefits of organic lip balms is that they are 100% natural! They are made from natural ingredients and are free from pesticides, chemicals and several other additives that are commonly found in conventional lip balms.

To give you a better idea of the hidden dangers lurking in your lip balm, we have discussed some ingredients used in lip balms that are harmful for your lips, and ultimately your health:

- **Mineral Oil** – Related to petroleum jelly, mineral oil contains neurotoxins, reproductive toxins, and carcinogens. This causes blackheads or breakouts around the lips. It also traps dirt and bacteria, which in turn blocks the absorption of minerals and vitamins into your lips.

- **Menthol, Phenol or Salicylic Acid** – These cause chemical burns due to which layers of your skin starts to peel off. This leaves your lips more chapped and therefore more exposed to environmental harm.

- **Petrolatum and Petroleum** – Studies show that they might cause cancer. They contain neurotoxins, reproductive toxins, and carcinogens, which causes skin irritation and allergies. In addition, petrolatum is a by-product of crude oil, which is a non-renewable resource. Therefore, there is a huge environmental impact involved as well.

- **Paraffin** –A by-product of crude oil, paraffin contains large quantities of dangerous compounds, such as lead, acetone, toluene, and benzene.

- **Lanolin** –Made from sheep's wool, chemicals are used to separate the wool and fat. It also can be contaminated by other plants.
- **Parabens** – It interferes with the hormones of the human body and is an endocrine disruptor. Parabens are also linked to organ toxicity, sterility, birth defects and cancer.
- **Phthalates** –Linked to birth defects, phthalates also increase the possibility of cell mutation and are known for being an endocrine disrupter.
- **Propylene Glycol** –Studies show it may cause damage to the liver, heart and the central nervous system.
- **Artificial Color, Scent, or Flavor** –These artificial ingredients can cause the skin to get irritated and burn.
- **Wheat and Soy** –Usually added as Vitamin E, wheat and soy are potential allergens for several people.

As you can see, by using a combination of these harmful ingredients lip balms are made commercially.

Who knew something so normal and small like lip balms could be dangerous? This is why organic lip balms are the way to go, as they are free of all sorts of chemicals and additives!

No Hidden Costs Involved

Yes, you may have to pay a premium price at the checkout counter for organic lip balms as opposed to conventional lip balms. And yes, due to this, you may think that the latter is the better option, considering it is cheaper.

However, first off, you must remember it does nothing to protect your lips. In addition to this, there are also hidden costs involved in the form of indirect taxes. So, you are actually paying pretty much the same amount for both, which is why you really do not need to compromise in quality.

How to Choose an Organic Lip Balm

Lip balms are perhaps the most ubiquitous lip care product on the market today. They can be bought from coffee shops, bookstores, grocery stores, and practically anywhere, that sells "impulse buy" items.

However, with thousands of lip balm brands available to choose from, it can be quite a daunting task to find the one best for you. Well, the variety available is overwhelming; there is no doubt about that, but if you keep a few things in mind, you will be able to find an organic lip balm that best suits your needs! Read on, as in the following paragraphs we will explain each of those things:

What Do You Need It For?

First, you must consider what you need the lip balm for. In other words, its application, for instance do you want to use it every day as an alternative to lip-gloss? Are you looking for medical treatment for your chapped and dry lips? Or maybe you want the super-protection you have always been longing for? Organic lip balms vary according to use, so make sure you know exactly what you want before buying!

The Type of Packaging You Want

Another important consideration to make is how you want to apply your lip balm. If you like dabbing it on with your fingers, a jar, or pot of organic lip balm is probably the right way to go. If you prefer squeezing the balm out, a tube is what you need. However, if you like sweeping it across your lips, a stick is definitely the best way to go.

Consider the Weather

To determine how often you need the lip balm to prevent your lips from drying and chapping, you will have to consider the weather and general climate in the place you live. For example, if you live in a location where the typical weather is cold and dry with a lot of sunlight, you will need to apply lip balm on a daily basis. On the other hand, if the weather is pleasant but not cold, humid and with limited sunlight, you will not need to use lip balm frequently.

Consider the Smell and Flavor

There are organic lip balms available in different fragrances and flavors. Some people love the fruity smell of lip balms while others find anything aromatic a bit too much to handle. Consider experimenting with a few organic lip balms as this would allow you to determine the flavors and scents which appeal to your senses.

Look For Super Friendly Oils

When buying an organic lip balm, always opt for the ones that contain almond oil and olive oil. If you are wondering why, that is because these particular oils are quite helpful in bringing back the natural oils of your lips, and thus give you clean, shiny, and healthy looking lips!

Pick a Balm with Benefits

There are organic lip balms that come with specific benefits as well. For example, balms that are made with high-grade oils, such as olive oil or tea tree oil, will moisturize and soothe your lips without leaving a greasy feeling. Similarly, lavender lip balms have a sweet herbal fragrance and are extremely effective at moisturizing the lips. Why not pick an organic lip balm that takes care of your lips while providing them some useful benefits?

Go For Lip Balms with Sunscreen

Lips are one of the most vulnerable places of the human body and can take quite a solar beating. This is why it's important that you look for organic lip balms that contain sun-blocking ingredients, so that your lips have optimum protection from the sun's harmful rays.

However, it is important to mention that some people are also sensitive to sunscreen, which could lead to even more chapping on their lips. Hence, if you notice any redness or itching, make sure you switch to an organic balm without sunscreen.

Treat the Problem

If you are dealing with severe dry, chapped, cracked, or peeling lips, do not hesitate in buying an organic medicated lip balm. It would not only soothe your lips from the irritation, but also get to the root of the problem, healing it quickly and effectively.

If you keep these considerations in mind, you will definitely be able to choose an organic lip balm that is right for you. However, do not compromise on quality just because good organic lip balms are usually expensive. While they may prove to be a little heavy on the wallet, the quality care they will provide your lips is totally worth the price!

6 Ingredients to Avoid in Lip Balms

Earlier on, we briefly discussed some of the most harmful ingredients used in lip balms. However, in this chapter, we will discuss 6 such ingredients in a lot more detail, so you can completely avoid the probability of applying harmful chemicals to your lips, that too, unknowingly!

As you probably may know, the skin on our lips is very thin, so much that ingredients are easily absorbed into the blood stream compared to other areas of our body. Throughout the day, lip balms are reapplied several times and you are likely to consume some of your applied lip balm by licking your lips.

That is why it is extremely important you make sure your lip balms are free from harmful ingredients. So, what are these ingredients? Several leading doctors and dermatologists recommend avoiding the following 6 ingredients in lip balms:

1. Synthetic Colors & Dyes (FD&C Green 3, Red 33, Blue 1, Yellow 5&6)

Derived from coal tar, FD&C color pigments contain heavy metal salts that leave toxins onto the skin. This causes severe skin irritation and sensitivity on your lips. According to studies, almost all FD&C colors are carcinogenic, therefore regular applications can lead to cancer!

2. Parabens (Butylparaben, Methylparaben, and More)

Parabens interfere with hormone functionality and are linked to reproductive toxicity and breast cancer. Moreover, it may also interfere with the reproductive functions of males, causing birth defects. In fact, in a recent study, it was found that Methylparaben blocks the breast cancer drug, tamoxifen.

3. Flavor & Fragrance

If you see 'flavor' or 'fragrance' written on the label of a lip balm, it is likely there will be hidden chemicals used to attain it. As a matter of fact, this is one of the biggest loopholes in FDA's federal law, as manufacturers are allowed to use almost any ingredient in their products under the word 'fragrance', that too without even naming the chemical.

Independent tests have shown that high levels of phthalates are found hiding in numerous products (including lip balms) under the word 'fragrance'. Phthalates are strong hormone disruptors and are linked to numerous conditions, such as allergies, pre-term births, reduced sperm counts in men, and asthma symptoms.

4. Chemical Sunscreens (Padimate O, Oxybenzone, Avobenzone, Octisalate, Octinoxate)

Chemical sunscreens penetrate the skin easily and could disrupt the hormone system of your body. One of the most common sunscreens, Oxybenzone, affects estrogen in the body and is also associated with endometriosis in women. That is why it is best you avoid lip balms with sunscreens. However, if you really do need a lip balm with sun protection, always purchase one with Zinc Oxide.

5. Petrolatum (Mineral Oil, Petroleum Jelly)

Over the past few years, the safety of petrolatum, regarding its use in cosmetic products has come into question. Because petrolatum is obtained from crude oil, it needs to be refined. However, toxic compounds are used in some refining methods. As a result, if the lip balm becomes contaminated during the manufacturing process, it is probable PAHs and other carcinogenic agents may affect it.

PAHs are associated with cancer and are potentially carcinogenic, which is why any traces of the chemical have to be removed after the refining process. In the European Union, there are strong regulations regarding the refining process, but unfortunately, no such regulations exist in the United States.

Moreover, petrolatum also creates an airtight barrier on the skin of your lips. Therefore, disrupting normal "breathing," and increasing absorption into the bloodstream.

6. Phenol

Because phenol is an effective bacteria killer, it has been used in several skin care products, such as whitening creams and lip balms. However, studies have shown it can also cause skin irritation, nervous system damage, as well as liver and kidney damage if absorbed by the skin regularly.

Therefore, whenever you see phenol listed on the ingredients of a particular lip balm, or any other skin care product for that matter, make sure you put down the lip balm and back away slowly!

As you can see, these 6 harmful ingredients in lip balms can cause a lot of problems in your body. That is why it is extremely important that you keep an eye out and avoid them when shopping around for lip balms!

Make Your Own Organic Lip Balm

Are you tired of using drugstore lip balms? If so, why don't you make your own organic lip balm at home? Lip balms are one of the easiest cosmetic products you can make at home. All you need to do is invest in the basic tools, and then you will be able to make organic lip balms for less than it costs at stores.

In this step-by-step guide, we will use a coconut lip balm recipe as an example. You will be amazed at how easy it is to make your own organic lip balm at home!

Things You Will Need:

- 1 ounce of jojoba
- 1 ounce of beeswax pellets
- 2 ounces of coconut oil
- 5 millimeters lime essential oil
- 24 lip balm tubes with lids
- 1 lip balm tube filling tray

- Spoon
- Glass-spouted measuring cup
- Kitchen scale
- Stovetop pot

Step #1: Prepare the Lip Balm Tubes

Place the empty lip balm tubes firmly onto the tray. According to this recipe, you will need at least 20 lip balm tubes, but this amount can differ from recipe to recipe. You should consider purchasing these tubes in bulk if you are looking to save some money.

Step #2: Measure and Melt the Beeswax

An easy way to measure the beeswax is by using a kitchen scale. Once you have measured the amount you require, melt the beeswax in a glass-measuring cup. However, remember you need to prevent the mixture from burning, so place the measuring cup in a shallow pot of boiling water. Keep stirring as the pellets begin to soften.

Step #3: Add the Coconut and Jojoba Oils

Once the pellets start melting, measure the amount of coconut and jojoba oil you require and pour it in the glass-measuring cup. By now, the coconut oil may be a soft or liquid paste, depending on the temperature inside your home. Continue to stir the mixture gently and once it is thoroughly combined, you should take it off the stove.

Step #4: Mix in the Essential Oil and Pour

Five millimeters of essential oils is equivalent to around 100 drops. You can use a slim graduated cylinder to easily measure the amount of essential oil you are mixing.

However, if you do not have one, simply count the drops. Though, it is not necessary that you have to be perfectly exact, it is recommended that you avoid adding more than the specified amount.

Once you have measured the essential oils, pour them into the hot oil mixture, and stir for a moment. Just before the mixture begins to cool, cautiously fill the tubes in the lip balm filling tray. Fill each tube to the top.

Step #5: Cool and Cap the Balm

After you filled the tubes with lip balm, leave the tray out for around 5 minutes, so that it can cool down a little. Then remove the tubes one at a time, and put the caps onto each. Although, they will appear to be solid quickly, you should wait at least 4 to 6 hours before using them.

Is Lip Balm Really Addictive?

This is one of the most common questions asked about lip balms. So, is it true or just another myth? Well, lip balms do not contain any ingredients or chemicals that make us psychologically addicted. However, several people claim they are addicted to using lip balms repeatedly throughout the day. Why is that so?

This is because most lip balms available today contain artificial ingredients that prolong the 'chapped effect', rather than curtailing it. Yes, the more you use such lip balms, the more your lips will be chapped! You have to admit, that is one devious way to ensure people keep buying your products.

These companies obtain harmful chemicals such as menthol, petrolatum, and phenol at cheap prices. These ingredients may create a pleasant tingling feel when you use the balm, but the sensation is actually nothing more than layers of your sensitive lip skin peeling off! As a result, your lips are left more exposed to the environmental factors that cause chapping.

Being out in the sun like this is another big concern, because the skin on our lips is more susceptible to developing severe cancer. Several dermatologists recommend using lip balms that contain sunscreen, so that the probability of such an incidence can completely be avoided.

They also recommend avoiding lip balms with added fragrances or flavors, because they may irritate the skin on your lips. Chapter 6, "Ingredients to Avoid in Lip Balms" details such ingredients.

Moving forward, are you aware of the difference between 'wax-based' and 'petroleum-based' lip balms? Well, some people believe wax-based products aren't as effective as petroleum-based ones. However, this opinion may vary depending on who you are talking to. On the other hand, several professionals 'claim' that using petroleum-based lip balms is safe 'enough', and does a great job trapping the moisture in our lips.

However, the truth is that just like the skin on our body needs to breath, so does the skin on our lips! Moreover, let's not forget petrolatum, petroleum jelly, and mineral oil, are all derived from crude oil. Even if you apply your lip balm in small amounts every day, most of it gets ingested, which adds up over time!

The European Union has banned several products based on petroleum. Moreover, while studies are being done to confirm the possibility of cancer due to these substances, the Food and Drug Administration (FDA) has hardly banned a few cosmetic products containing petroleum. The Manager of the Dallas International Dermal Institute, Jennifer Loza, stated:

"Petroleum-based products offer a sense a false hydration and can lead to irritation. This cheap ingredient is still found in cosmetic preparations however should be avoided as it is highly comedogenic (doesn't allow for lips to breath). Better ingredients for the lips include shea butter, avocado, cocoa butter, wheat germ and Vitamin E as they actually provide a number of benefits, including conditioning and moisturizing the skin."

This means lip balms containing petroleum are actually harmful for your health, particularly when synthetic ingredients are used. This is why it is best you avoid them. However, sadly many people are not aware of the consequences involved because of their use.

So, what is the solution to this problem? Should you use other lip balms or completely avoid using them for good? Well, the answer is quite simple. Your best bet is using an organic lip balm, because they are free from all sorts of questionable chemicals, and are only made from natural ingredients.

Always remember to check the label before buying lip balms. Even if it says it's organic. It will save you from a lot of 'chapping' troubles ahead!

How to Deal With Lip Balm Addiction

As mentioned above, lip balm really isn't addictive, and neither is there anything in them that drives us to be psychologically dependent on them. However, if you become addicted to lip balm, it is extremely important you reduce the amount you are applying every day.

The main concern though is how, right? Whenever you do not have your lip balm with you, it's a big problem. You are addicted to it and can't help but getting your hands on some to nourish your lips.

Nevertheless, that does not necessarily mean there is no remedy to this uncontrollable addiction. We have discussed a few helpful tips below that will help you overcome your lip balm addiction as soon as possible.

Use Organic Lip Balms

There are many questionable ingredients used in both wax-based and petroleum based lip balms that prolong the chapping effect on your lips. As a result, most people tend to use these lip balms more than often to moisturize their lips. However, this too, does nothing more than aggravate the problem even further!

That is why several dermatologists and doctors recommend you use organic lip balms. Not only are they free from all sorts of harmful chemicals and ingredients used in most lip balms today, they are made from natural ingredients, which will protect and treat your chapped lips effectively, minus the damage.

Know about the Sun's Rays

The skin on your lips burns too, especially when they are chapped. In fact, there is a lot more at stake than just simple irritation or burning, because the skin on our lips is more prone to developing severe forms of cancer.

According to Todd Perkins, a renowned dermatologist in Washington, D.C, these cancers spread quicker on the lips than any other part of our body. That is why it's extremely important you apply sunscreen on both your lips. If possible, try to purchase and use safe organic lip balms with SPF sunscreen protection.

Is it the Product or the Behavior?

You need to determine what's causing the addiction. Is it the product or the behavior? While lip balms may not cause physiological dependence, we can be addicted to it, leading us to making some lifestyle changes.

For example, people who love darker shades of lipstick will always find themselves purchasing darker colors of clothing as well. As such, they won't even wear bright colored clothes during summer. In this scenario, it is important you reduce the amount of lip balm you apply.

This can be done by reaching for your water bottle whenever you feel compelled to apply lip balms. Besides, most people do not have enough water, and the hydration will help your lips as well as your mind and body.

However, if it's your lip balm, we recommend replacing it right away. Always use organic lip balms, because they are natural, healthy and extremely beneficial for your lips.

How to Treat Chapped Lips Effectively?

Chapped and dry lips are a sign of winter and dryness. While you bundle up extra layers of clothing during these months, it does not change the fact that your lips are still exposed to the sun, and cold and dry air.

Since our lips have the thinnest layers of skin compared to other parts of the body, they are more likely to dry out. This can dehydrate your lips, leaving them with no moisture whatsoever. Eventually, they develop cracks and splits.

However, this time, things can be different! All you need to do is protect your lips with organic lip balms. They provide a barrier between the weather and your delicate skin, so your lips are never left bare. Nevertheless, there are a few other tips you should keep in mind as well. These include:

Avoid Licking Your Lips

As the weather becomes colder and the air drier, people tend to lick their lips more than often. However, the truth is that licking your lips does nothing more than making your chapping worse. That is because the saliva evaporates and leaves the lips even drier and irritable than before.

Another common mistake most people make is to bite, scrub, and peel skin flakes off; the result of chapped lips. Remember, the skin of your lips is already very thin and picking at it will only cause severe discomfort and bleeding. As a result, the healing process slows down and will lead to a cold sore or infection.

Apply Balm Early & Often

The key to preventing your lips from becoming flaky and cracked is to apply lip balm early and often. Since most people tend to sleep with their mouths open, it causes their lips to dry out almost completely. Therefore, it is best you wear a thick layer of balm on your lips at bedtime.

By doing so, you will be less likely to wake up with chapped lips. Moreover, always keep your organic lip balm handy. Keep one near your bed, one in the car, and one at your workplace for convenience.

However, don't go overboard and apply more than you require. Too much of anything is bad, remember? It is also recommended that you drink plenty of water to fight dehydration, because it is also one of the leading causes of chapped lips!

Be Cautious With Lip Balms

Some lip balms do a lot more harm than good. That is because the ingredients used are cheap and often harmful, causing irritation and dryness. Always take a close look at the label before purchasing organic lip balms to ensure there are no dangerous chemicals or substances included.

Some examples of such ingredients include petrolatum, menthol, chemical sunscreens etc. Additionally, it is recommended you avoid lip balms that come in little jars or pots, because applying balm with your fingers isn't really as hygienic as through a tube applicator.

So, keep these tips in mind, and treating your chapped lips shouldn't really be a problem!

25 Best Organic Lip Balm Recipes

Ever tried making your own organic lip balm at home? If not, you will be surprised at how much fun it can be. What's even better is that once you get it right, you will be able to make organic lip balms for less than the ones available in the markets.

So, are you ready? In this chapter, we have discussed 10 simple yet effective organic lip balm recipes to get you started!

1. Silky Smooth Lip Balm

Ingredients:

- 2 Tsp Olive Oil
- ½ Tsp Cocoa Butter or Shea Butter
- ½ Tsp Beeswax Pellets or Grated Beeswax
- ½ Tsp Honey
- Any organic flavored oil to taste

Instructions:

In a microwave-safe bowl, mix the first four ingredients together thoroughly, and microwave the mixture until it melts entirely. (You can also heat the bowl in a pan of water on the stovetop).

Then, add the organic flavored oil and stir well. Leave the mixture to cool for about five minutes and stir once again. Now, set it aside to cool completely. Once it's cooled, pour the mixture into lip balm tubes and put on the lids.

2. Vitamin E Honey Lip Balm

Ingredients:

- 3 Ounces Almond Oil
- ½ Ounces Beeswax Pellets or Beeswax
- 2 Tsp Honey
- 1-4 Drops Essential Oil
- 1 Vitamin E Capsule (as a preservative)

Instructions:

In a microwave-safe bowl, mix the beeswax and almond oil thoroughly, and microwave the mixture for a few minutes until it melts entirely. Then, stir the mixture until the wax melts. Once it does, remove the mixture from the heat, add the essential oil and honey, and stir thoroughly.

Squeeze the contents of the Vitamin E capsule into the mixture and stir again. Now, set it aside to cool completely. Once it's cooled, pour the mixture into lip balm tubes and tighten the lids.

3. Cocoa Butter Minty Lip Balm

Ingredients:

- 1 ½ Parts Grated Beeswax
- 1 ½ Parts Cocoa Butter
- 3 Parts (Edible) Vegetable Oil of your preference
- Peppermint or/and Spearmint organic flavored oil

Instructions:

In a microwave, or over a double boiler on the stove, melt the beeswax and cocoa butter carefully and slowly. Once it melts, add the vegetable oil, and stir well. Then, add peppermint or spearmint organic flavored oils (you can also add both) one drop at a time.

Set aside to cool before you pour it into the lip balm tubes and place and tighten the lids. If you want to make the lip balm softer, add more vegetable oil. To make the lip balm harder, add more beeswax.

4. Hemp Oil Lip Balm

Ingredients:

- 3 Tbsp Coconut Oil
- 1 Tbsp Sunflower Oil
- 1 Tbsp Castor Oil
- 1 Tbsp Hemp Seed Oil
- 1 Tbsp Honey
- 1 Tbsp Beeswax
- Any essential oil to taste

Instructions:

Melt the coconut oil and beeswax together, using the microwave or stovetop. Once it melts, add honey, and continue heating a little. Then, stirring consistently, add castor oil and sunflower oil.

By now, you will notice the mixture is thickening. Add the essential oil and hemp oil and stir until it thickens. Hemp oil lip balms are best used when stored in a small jar or pot.

5. Sweet Lip Balm

Ingredients:

- 1 Tsp Honey
- 2 Tsp Beeswax
- 7 Tsp Sweet Almond Oil or Jojoba Oil or Castor Oil
- 1/8 Tsp organic flavored oil

Instructions:

In a pan over the stove's low heat, melt the beeswax and the oil of your choice together. Once the beeswax melts, take it off the stove, add the honey and whisk it all thoroughly. Then, add in the organic flavored oils, stir the mixture and set it aside to cool completely.

When the mixture cools down, pour it into the lip balm tubes and put on the lids. Since the recipe usually results in a more glossy consistency, consider adding a little more beeswax in order to make it harder. Another ½ tsp should do the trick!

6. Healing & Nourishing Lip Balm

Ingredients:

- 1 Tbsp Shaved Cocoa Butter
- 1 Tbsp + 1 Tsp Shaved Beeswax
- 3 Tbsp Coconut Oil
- 1 Drop Peppermint Essential Oil

Instructions:

Over the stove, or in the microwave, melt the first three ingredients together. Once everything melts entirely, whisk the mixture thoroughly. Then, remove off the heat and pour the mixture into lip balm tubes and place and tighten the lids. leave the tubes out to cool overnight.

7. Glossy Lip Balm

Ingredients:

- 2 Ounces + 1 Tbsp Organic Extra Virgin Coconut Oil
- 1.5 Tbsp Vitamin E Essential Oil
- 2 Ounces Beeswax
- (Optional) 25 Drops peppermint or vanilla essential oil for fragrance

Instructions:

In a bowl, place the beeswax, coconut oil and Vitamin E oil. Then, fill a pan with water, place it on the stove, and bring it to a boil. Be cautious you do not place the bowl right away, because the heat may cause the bowl to crack.

Once the water is about to boil, place the bowl onto the pan and melt the oils. You should have a nice golden liquid once all the oils have melted (the beeswax will take the longest amount of time).

If you want to add fragrances, add peppermint or vanilla essential oils while the balm is still over the heat. Add a few drops at a time because some oils are stronger than the others. Once the balm is sufficiently scented, pour it into the lip balm tubes, and let it cool.

8. Beeswax Lip Balm

Ingredients:

- 1 Tbsp Coconut Oil
- 2 Tbsp Beeswax

Instructions:

Over a double boiler, melt both the ingredients together. Once the mixture melts entirely, pour it into lip balm tubes and put on the lids. Set aside to cool fully.

9. Cherry Grape Seed Lip Balm

Ingredients:

- 2 Tbsp Beeswax (Grated)
- 1-2 Cups Grape Seed Oil
- 3 Drops Vitamin E Oil
- 10 Drops Organic Cherry Flavoring Oil
- Organic Red Cosmic Dye

Instructions:

In a glass-measuring cup, add the grape seed oil and beeswax. Then, wrap the cup using plastic wrap, place the cup over a pan on the stove, and start heating the oil. Make sure you stir, and continue heating, until the beeswax melts.

Carefully add the organic red dye to the mixture until you reach the desired shade. You have to stir the mixture gently in order to ensure the dye evenly distributes. Add in the vitamin E and flavoring oils and stir the mixture thoroughly. Once the lip balm is properly mixed, pour the mixture into ¼- oz containers and leave it to cool and harden.

10. Nutmeg & Mandarin Luscious Lip Balm

Ingredients:

- 2 Tbsp Sunflower Oil
- 1 Tbsp Olive Oil
- 1 Tbsp Beeswax or Beeswax Pastilles
- 1 Tbsp Mango Butter (You can also use shea butter)
- 5 Drops Nutmeg Essential Oil
- 2 Drops Vitamin E Oil (Optional)
- 15 Drops Mandarin Essential Oil

Instructions:

Place the double boiler over the stove, and boil water in the bottom of the saucepan. In the meantime, cut the beeswax, and add it along with the butter and oils into a glass jug.

Once the water reaches boiling point, place the glass jug in the top of the double boiler allow it to melt gently. When the mixture fully melts, remove the jug from the stove, add in the vitamin E and essential oil, and stir gently.

Allow the mixture to cool slightly before you pour it into the lip balm tubes. Let it cool completely before you put the lids on and that is about it!

11. Coconut Mango Butter Lip Balm

Ingredients:

- 1 Tbsp Mango Butter
- 1 Tbsp and Tsp Beeswax Pastilles
- 1 Tbsp Coconut Oil
- ½ Tbsp Castor Oil
- ½ Tbsp Jojoba Oil
- 1 Tbsp Olive Oil (Calendula Infused)

Instructions:

Add all the ingredients into a glass-measuring cup, and place it into a pan or double boiler containing a few inches of water. Allow the water to heat gently, as you do not want any boiling or steam going on.

Continue heating and stir gently, until the beeswax pastilles and mango butter have melted completely. Then, remove the cup from the heat and pour the lip balm into lip balm tubes, containers, or tins. Let it cool before you place the lids on.

12.Minty Chocolate Lip Balm

Ingredients:

- 2 Tbsp Sweet Almond Oil
- 1 Tbsp Avocado Oil
- 1 Tbsp Cocoa Butter
- 1 Tbsp and Tsp Beeswax Pellets
- 2 Drops Vitamin E Oil
- 12-15 Drops Peppermint Essential Oil

Instructions:

Add the beeswax, cocoa butter, avocado oil, and almond oil to your glass-measuring cup and place it in the top of your double boiler. Heat it gently until the contents are completely melted.

Then remove the double boiler from the stove, add peppermint essential oil and vitamin E oil into the mixture, and stir gently. Immediately pour the lip balm into lip balm contains, preferably 3 x ½ oz. jars or tins. Let the mixture cool before you apply the lids on.

13.Coconut Oil Lip Balm

Ingredients:

- 1 Tsp Olive Oil or Red Palm Oil
- 1 Tbsp Coconut Oil
- 1 Tbsp Beeswax

Instructions:

Add the beeswax, olive oil or red palm oil, and coconut oil into a glass-measuring cup and place it into the double boiler. Heat the contents gently and stir often, until the wax and oils are completely melted.

Once the mixture melts, stir it thoroughly. Then, pour the lip balm into tubes, storage container, or jar, whichever your preference. Put it away to cool for a few hours and its ready to use!

14. Warm Honey & Vanilla Lip Balm

Ingredients:

- 3 Tbsp Beeswax
- 2 Tbsp Shea Butter
- 2 Tbsp Sweet Almond Oil
- 1 ½ Tbsp Organic Honey
- ½ Tsp Vanilla Oil

Instructions:

Add the shea butter, beeswax, and almond oil into a glass-measuring cup, and place it into a double boiler over a low heat. Stir continuously until all the ingredients melt and blend completely.

Then, remove the double boiler from the heat, and add in the vanilla oil and organic honey. Whisk well using a chopstick, or small whisk, and distribute the honey evenly throughout the mixture.

Pour the lip balm into tins or tubes and allow them to cool until they become hard. Once it does, apply the lids, and store or use as you please! However, when storing, make sure the lip balm is kept away from heat.

15.Peppermint Lip Balm

Ingredients:

- 2 Tbsp Carrier Oil
- 1 Tbsp Beeswax Pellets
- 8 Drops Peppermint Essential Oil
- Organic Lipstick Shavings (for a touch of tint)

Instructions:

Put in the beeswax and carrier oil into a glass jar, close the lid, and heat it gently in a double boiler or pot with water, until the wax melts completely. Once melted, remove from the heat and stir the mixture thoroughly.

Then, add the pepper essential oil using a dropper and make sure you keep it to eight drops, as adding any more would be unnecessary. If you prefer your lip balm to be tinted, stir in some organic lipstick shavings, until you achieve the desired color.

Finally, pour the mixture into containers or lip balm tubes, and leave it to cool for a few hours until it hardens.

16.Luscious Lavender Lip Balm

Ingredients:

- 4 Tbsp Jojoba, Olive, or Almond Oil
- 1 Tbsp Beeswax Pearls or Grated Beeswax
- ¼ Tsp Vitamin E Oil
- 1 Tsp Honey
- 1 Tsp Cocoa Powder (optional)
- 7 Drops Lavender Essential Oil

Instructions:

Heat the honey, oils, and beeswax in a stainless steel bowl or pot. Make sure to heat it on a very low heat using a double boiler. Stir gently, and continue doing so until the beeswax melts completely.

Once melted, remove the mixture from the heat, and immediately add in the cocoa powder, vitamin E oil, and essential oil. Using a whisk, thoroughly whisk the contents, and continue whisking as you add the honey.

When the honey incorporates, pour the lip balm into a container or lip balm tubes, and allow it to set for at least 3-4 hours before using.

(**Tip:** If you do not want to rush to transferring the lip balm into the tubes, let the cup/bowl remain over the double boiler)

17.Super Moisturizing Lip Balm

Ingredients:

- 3 Tsp Organic Coconut Oil (Unrefined)
- 2 Tsp Cosmetic Grade Beeswax Pastilles
- 1 Tsp Shea Butter
- 10 Drops Tangerine Essential Oil
- 10 Drops Peppermint Essential Oil

Instructions:

Combine all the ingredients in a glass-measuring cup or bowl, and put it in a double boiler on a low heat. Stir the mixture gently, and continue doing so until the shea butter and beeswax melts.

Once melted, remove the glass-measuring cup or bowl from the heat, and pour the lip balm into tubes or containers using a funnel. Leave it undisturbed for about 20-30 minutes, so that it cools and sets down.

18.Essential Lip Balm

Ingredients:

- 3 Tbsp Beeswax
- 2 Tbsp Organic Coconut Oil
- 1 Tbsp Shea Butter
- 1 Tbsp Cocoa Butter
- 10 Drops Lavender Essential Oil
- 20 Drops Peppermint Essential Oil

Instructions:

Add all the oils and butters into a glass-measuring jar, and put it into a double boiler or pan with boiling water. Gently stir the ingredients as they melt, and continue doing so until they are properly combined.

Once the wax completely melts, remove the glass-measuring jar from the heat and let it sit for about 3 minutes. Then, add the peppermint and lavender essential oils but make sure they do not exceed the specified amount. Using a funnel can be particularly helpful.

Pour the lip balm into tubes, jars, or containers, set it aside to cool down, and your essential lip balm is finally ready to use!

19.Vanilla Lip Balm

Ingredients:

- 2 Tbsp Organic Coconut Oil
- 1 ½ Tbsp Beeswax
- 1 Tbsp Shea Butter
- 1 Tbsp Sweet Almond Oil
- ½ Tsp Vanilla Essential Oil

Instructions:

Add the beeswax, shea butter, sweet almond oil, and organic coconut oil, into a glass-measuring cup. Then, over a double boiler, or pan of water, heat the ingredients and whisk together.

Once it has completely melted, remove the glass-measuring cup from the stove, and leave it to cool for a few minutes. Use a pipette or funnel to pour the lip balm into tubes and apply the lids on. Put the lip balm away to set for approximately 12 hours before use!

20.Luscious Lemon Lip Balm

Ingredients:

- 1 Part Shea Butter
- 1 Part Beeswax Pellets
- 3-5 Drops Lemon Essential Oil

Instructions:

Place a pan or double boiler with over medium heat. In the meantime, add the shea butter, avocado oil, and beeswax into a glass-measuring cup or jar. Once the water reaches boiling point, place it in the water, and stir gently as the beeswax slowly melts.

Once it has completely melted, remove the glass-measuring cup, or jar from the heat, and leave it to cool. In about 10 minutes or so, the lip balm will begin to show signs of solidification.

Immediately add the essential oil and stir thoroughly. Using a funnel, pour in the lip balm into tubes or containers, and leave it to harden.

(**Note:** It is very important you know that some citrus essential oils are phototoxic. Therefore, if you live in a climate where sunlight is the standard, replace the lemon essential oil with peppermint or lavender for an equally effective and luscious lip balm)

21.Rosy Rose Lip Balm

Ingredients:

- 2 Tbsp Sweet Almond or Coconut Oil
- 2 Tsp Beeswax
- ¼ Tsp Organic Lipstick (Grated)
- 1 Vitamin E capsule
- 5-6 Drops Rose Essential Oil

Instructions:

In a glass-measuring cup, add the beeswax along with coconut or sweet almond oil. Then, place it over a pan or double boiler with water, and stir gently as the beeswax slowly melts.

Once it melts completely, add the grated lipstick if you prefer a little color in your lip balm. Stir gently, and continue doing so, as you add the Rose essential oil into the mixture.

Puncture a Vitamin E capsule and add as well. Mix thoroughly using a whisk, until all the ingredients are properly combined. Once done, pour the lip balm into tubes, and set aside to cool before using!

22.Tinted Lip Balm

Ingredients:

- 2 Tbsp Coconut Oil
- 1 Tbsp Cocoa Butter or Shea Butter
- 1 Tbsp Beeswax Pastilles
- Organic Lip Stick (grated)
- Essential Oil (Whichever you prefer)

Instructions:

Melt the cocoa or shea butter, beeswax, and coconut oil in a glass-measuring cup over a pan of simmering water, and stir gently until all the ingredients have completely melted.

Once melted, remove the glass-measuring cup from the heat, and add in the essential oil and organic lipstick. Stir gently because it is extremely important the ingredients mix in properly.

Then, using a funnel, pour the lip balm into containers or tubes, whichever is your preference. Leave the lip balm for a few hours, so that it can cool and harden before use.

23.Lavender Mint Lip Balm

Ingredients:

- 2 Tbsp Beeswax Pastilles
- 2 Tbsp Coconut Oil
- 2 Tbsp Shea Butter
- 12 Drops Peppermint Essential Oil
- 8 Drops Lavender Essential Oil

Instructions:

Add the beeswax, shea butter, and coconut oil in a glass-measuring cup, and place it in a pot or double boiler with simmering water. Keep the heat low, and stir gently. Continue doing so until the ingredients have melted completely.

Once the ingredients are fully combined, turn the heat off, and let the glass-measuring cup with the mixture cool slightly. It is important to keep the mixture in hot water, because it will begin to harden quickly!

Then, add the peppermint and lavender essential oils into the mixture, and stir thoroughly. Using a funnel, immediately pour the lip balm into tubes or container and put it away to cool and harden.

24.Coco-Rosey Lip Balm

Ingredients:

- 2 Tbsp Coconut Oil
- ¼ Tbsp Vitamin E Oil
- 1 Tbsp Cocoa Butter (Grated)
- 1 Tbsp dried rosebuds
- 3 Drops Rose Essential Oil

Instructions:

Melt the coconut oil in a glass-measuring cup on a very low heat. Once the oil becomes liquid, add the roses, stir thoroughly, and let it steep (again) on a very low heat for about an hour.

Then, strain the mixture into another bowl using a cheesecloth or fine-mesh sieve. With a clean cloth, wipe out the glass-measuring cup, and pour the mixture back in again. Make sure the heat is kept very low!

Add in the cocoa butter, and stir gently, until it completely combines with the mixture. Once it mixes properly, remove the glass-measuring cup from the heat, and add the rose essential oil and vitamin E oil.

Mix well, and pour the lip balm into tubes or containers and allow it to set for about 2-3 hours.

25.All-Natural Lip Balm

Ingredients:

- 4 Tbsp Coconut Oil
- 2 Tbsp Beeswax Pellets
- ½ Tsp Vitamin E Oil
- Essential Oils Of Your Choice

Instructions:

In a glass-measuring cup, add the coconut oil and beeswax, and put it in a double boiler on low heat. Stir gently, and continue doing so, until both the ingredients have melted together completely.

Once they have melted, remove the glass-measuring cup from the heat, and add Vitamin E oil. Stir the mixture thoroughly, and then add the essential oils of your preference, about 20-30 drops. Pour the lip balm into containers or tubes, and set it aside to cool and harden!

There you have it. 25 of the best organic lip balm recipes, all in one place! So, what are you waiting for? Try them out, and provide your lips the best protection and care during winters!

18 Unique Uses of Lip Balm (Bonus Chapter)

Interestingly enough, lip balms can be used on a lot more than just your lips. They can be used to keep other areas moisturized and looking great. In some cases, they can do a lot more.

Thanks to their soothing formula and tacky consistency, lip balms are actually handy for loads of other beauty and household uses. And the best part about all this is they can be taken with you wherever you go. That is because their size allows you to throw one in your pocket or bag when you are heading out.

In this bonus chapter, you will be acquainted with 20 unique and clever uses of lip balms other than healing chapped lips:

1. Stop Bleeding from Minor Cuts

Ever cut yourself while shaving? The next time it happens, ditch the embarrassing piece of toilet paper on your face or neck, and apply a coat of lip balm instead. Turns out its moisturizing ingredients are a great way to heal cuts on other parts of your body as well.

2. Moisturize Elbows & Knees

Elbows and knees tend to have the driest and roughest skin on the entire body. However, you can soften them effectively with the moisturizing lip balms.

3. Lubricate Zippers

Sometimes the zippers of your jackets or backpacks can be stuck and make getting dressed or packing your bag a tougher task then it needs to be. Therefore, try applying some lip balm! The natural oils can help lubricate the zippers, ensuring they run smoother.

4. Shine Your Shoes

Are your shoes looking a little dull? If so, apply a little lip balm on your shoes and polish them using a dry cloth, making it an easy and quick way to get a shoeshine.

5. Sooth Rashes

Did you know that lip balms could be used to soothe rashes and dry skin? Thanks to its high Vitamin E and Aloe Vera content, lip balms will repair and soothe your skin effectively and quickly.

6. Repair Scratched CD's

Rub a thin coat of lip balm across the scratches on your CD and wipe it off using a soft clean cloth. The natural oils will prevent your CD from skipping and ensure they run smoother.

7. Protect Your Entire Face

Rubbing a little lip balm on your face will provide a strong barrier between your face and whatever you want to protect it from.

8. Use as a Base for Make-Up

Many ladies use lip balms as a base with their makeup or eye shadow. Lip balms can be used to make a foundation or cream-shadow.

9. Keep Your Shoes Tied

To prevent your shoes from becoming undone, simply apply a coat of lip balm on the strings and tie the knot. This works great on ice skates as well!

10. Groom Your Eyebrows

If you are out of brow gel, or just aren't in the mood to buy some, gently tap a little lip balm along your eyebrows while you brush them into place. The consistency of lip balms will prevent your eyebrows from straying without feeling tacky.

11. Stop High Heel Chaffing

The waxiness of lip balms provides a great barrier for your skin against the friction of painful and new shoes. Therefore, whenever you feel the burn, simply rub a little lip balm onto the area and you are good to go!

12. For Your Nose

Dry skin surrounding your nose is quite common in winter. The area around the nose tends to dry and become rough. However, did you know the moisturizing oils in lip balms can help soothe the dry skin surrounding your nose? All you have to do is rub a little onto your nostrils and your skin will thank you!

13. Hammer & Nail Help

At times, it can be difficult hammering or screwing a nail or screw into the wall. By applying a little lip balm to them before hammering or screwing, you can get it into the wall without the need of much force.

14. Track Grease

Are the tracks on your bedroom window or medicine cabinet giving you a hard time? If so, use a little lip balm to grease them. Before you know it, they will be as good as new!

15. Remove a Stubborn Ring

We all know oil, butter and moisturizers are great to get a ring off a finger. However, did you know lip balms can also be used to remove those stubborn rings? Simply apply a little lip balm on your finger and around the ring in order slide it effortlessly off.

16. Prevent a Light Bulb from Sticking

When lighting is exposed to outdoor elements, they usually get stuck and become hard to remove. Therefore, before you set the light bulb into the socket, apply a little lip balm to its thread. As a result, you will be able to remove it later on with ease.

17. Condition Your Nails

Apply a little lip balm to your nails and cuticles, and leave it for a few minutes. Then, using an orange stick, gently push the cuticles down. The moisturizing content of lip balms conditions your nails and softens the cuticles.

18. Protect Your Skin from Hair Dye

Hair dyes usually strain the skin. However, you can protect your skin from hair dyes effectively by applying a little lip balm around your hairline.

As you can see, a small tube of lip balm does a lot more than just healing your chapped lips. Isn't it amazing? Try these! You will be surprised at how effective these tips are!

Final Words

And with that last chapter, we come to the end of the eBook. It's been a really great journey and we are glad to have offered as much information as we could.

We hope you have enjoyed the eBook and have found a lot of great information in it. We wanted to ensure you learned as much as you could about organic lip balm, what it can do, how you can use and make it, its benefits, and what you should stay away from.

While we have carefully gathered all the information, we strongly advise you get in touch with your doctor or dermatologist before making any major changes regarding your lip's care.

Additionally, if you buy organic lip balms from stores, we strongly advise you keep an eye out for any harmful ingredients. On the other hand, if you are making your own organic lip balm, ensure that you follow the mentioned guidelines so you do not mess up!

Now that you know about organic lips balms, you no longer have to reach for the harmful chemical-filled lip balms on your supermarket aisles. Not only are they free from all sorts of harmful chemicals; they are also made from natural, healing ingredients that treat your chapped lips effectively. We assure you nothing can rejuvenate, nourish, and protect your lips as naturally as organic lip balms! So what are you waiting for? It is time to get out there are buy/make some organic lip balm and moisturize your life!

Until next time, good luck and good-bye!